LYMPHEDEMA AND LIPEDEMA BAKING GUIDE

A Guide to Transform Your Health with Lymph-Friendly Baking

Kimberly Williams J.

TABLE OF CONTENTS

The goal of this guide is to give readers with practical and efficient treatments for lymphatic health, with an emphasis on disorders like lymphedema and lipedema. We aim to improve overall quality of life while managing these chronic disorders by providing scientifically validated recipes and insights on the importance of adequate nutrition.

Understanding Lymphedema and Lipedema.

Lymphedema and lipedema are two different yet related lymphatic diseases. Lymphedema occurs when lymphatic vessels are injured or clogged, causing fluid buildup and swelling in the arms and legs. Lipedema, on the other hand, is defined by abnormal fat formation, which is frequently disproportionate to weight growth and results in painful and swollen limbs. Both situations can have a substantial impact on daily operations and necessitate specialized management strategies.

Causes and Symptoms

The causes of lymphedema differ depending on whether it is primary (genetic) or secondary (due to injury, surgery, or radiation therapy). Common symptoms include prolonged swelling, tight skin, weight, discomfort, and recurring infections. Similarly, lipedema develops as a result of genetic and hormonal abnormalities, resulting in distinct patterns of fat distribution and discomfort. Common symptoms include heavy and sore limbs, trouble fitting into clothing, and heightened sensitivity to touch.

The Importance of Nutrition in Management

Adequate diet is essential for controlling lymphedema and lipedema. Balanced diets high in important vitamins, minerals, antioxidants, and anti-inflammatory chemicals aid to reduce inflammation, enhance circulation, and promote tissue healing. Furthermore, keeping a healthy body weight and avoiding excessive salt consumption might help prevent subsequent issues from fluid retention. This article will go over several food options and meal plans designed to improve lymphatic function and efficiently manage associated symptoms.

Chapter 1: Principles of Lymph-Friendly Baking

Understanding the fundamentals of a lymph-friendly diet is critical for people seeking to treat lymphedema and lipedema. A lymph-friendly diet attempts to reduce inflammation, boost immunological function, and improve waste elimination through the lymphatic system. Focusing on whole foods, balanced macronutrients, and appropriate hydration promotes lymph flow and lowers the likelihood of problems.

The key principles of a lymph-friendly diet are:

1. Consuming high-quality proteins, including lean meats, fish, eggs, legumes, nuts, seeds, and plant-based protein sources.

2. Opting for complex carbs such as fruits, vegetables, whole grains, and starchy tubers.

3. Include lots of fiber-rich meals like leafy greens, cruciferous vegetables, berries, and legumes.

4. Avocados, olive oil, fatty fish, nuts, and seeds all contain beneficial fats.

5. Limiting processed foods, refined sugars, saturated and trans fats, and excessive sodium.

Important Ingredients for Lymphedema and Lipedema

Incorporating specific components proven to enhance lymphatic health will help you make lymph-friendly baked goods. The key elements are:

1. Leafy green veggies are high in chlorophyll, folate, and antioxidants, which help with detoxification and immunity. Examples include spinach, kale, collard greens and Swiss chard.

2. Cruciferous veggies: High in sulphur compounds, cruciferous vegetables promote liver detoxification and have anti-inflammatory effects. Examples include broccoli, Brussels sprouts, cabbage, and cauliflower.

3. Antioxidant-rich fruits are high in flavonoids, carotenoids, and polyphenols, which help to protect against oxidative stress and free radical damage. Blueberries, strawberries, raspberries, and apples are a few examples.

4. Omega-3 fatty acids: Flaxseeds, walnuts, chia seeds, and fatty fish such as salmon and mackerel are high in omega-3 fatty acids, which are necessary for inflammation reduction and cardiovascular health improvement.

5. Probiotic-rich fermented foods: By increasing gut microbial diversity and digestive health, probiotics help to boost immune function and reduce

inflammation. Yoghurt, kefir, sauerkraut, and tempeh are a few examples.

6. Plant-based proteins such as beans, lentils, chickpeas, and tofu provide a diversity of amino acids while reducing inflammation.

7. Prebiotic fibers: Prebiotic fibers feed the healthy bacteria in our gastrointestinal tract, promoting better digestion and nutritional absorption. Examples include oats, bananas, Jerusalem artichokes, and leeks.

Alternative Baking Recipes for Healthier Options

Substitution approaches are required when adapting classic baking recipes to include more lymph-friendly foods. Here are some recommendations for healthier ingredient replacements:

1. Replace white flour with whole grain flours like spelt, buckwheat, or almond flour for more fibre and minerals.

2. Using unsweetened applesauce instead of butter or oil increases moisture and flavour while decreasing calorie intake.

3. Swapping granulated sugar for natural sweeteners such as raw honey, pure maple syrup, or dates improves taste while reducing blood sugar rises.

4. Using mashed ripe bananas or blended prunes in place of additional sugars increases sweetness and fiber content.

5. Experimenting with alternative milks, such as almond milk, cashew milk, or hemp milk, provides fewer calories and more nutrients than cow's milk.

6. Choosing unrefined sea salt over table salt increases trace nutrients and enhances flavour characteristics.

7. Adding herbs and spices like turmeric, ginger, rosemary, thyme, and oregano has powerful anti-inflammatory properties while also improving flavour.

Tools and Equipment.

Making lymph-friendly baked goodies is easier and more pleasurable when you have the proper tools and equipment. Some recommended items are:

1. Measuring cups and spoons: Measuring ingredients correctly guarantees consistent outcomes.

2. Mixing bowls come in a variety of sizes, allowing you to mix little batches or big volumes.

3. Hand mixer or stand mixer: Effectively combines wet and dry materials.

4. Silicon spatulas are useful for scraping down the sides of mixing basins to ensure level mixing.

5. Rolling pin: Used to roll out dough and shape cookies.

6. Nonstick baking sheets: Reduces sticking and makes cleanup easier.

7. A cooling rack allows baked items to properly cool after being removed from the oven.

8. Food processor or blender: Ideal for crushing nuts, seeds, and pulverising dried fruits.

9. Grater: Used to zest citrus peels and finely grate vegetables.

10. Kitchen scale: Accurately weighs materials, especially for gluten-free baking.

Understanding the foundations of lymph-friendly baking, selecting acceptable ingredients, and using proper substitutions and equipment will allow you to create tasty and healthy baked items that promote lymphatic health.

Breakfast Delights

1. Green Goddess Breakfast Bowl:
Ingredients:
For the basis:
1/2 cup cooked quinoa or brown rice.
A handful of spinach or kale, roughly chopped
1/4 cup of roasted sweet potato cubes.
1/4 cup cherry tomatoes, halved

For toppings:
1/2 avocado, cut.
1/4 cup crumbled feta cheese.
2 tablespoons sunflower seeds.
1/4 cup chopped fresh herbs (parsley, cilantro, and dill).
For the Green Goddess Dressing:
1/2 avocado, pitted and peeled.
1/4 cup of fresh parsley leaves.
1/4 cup fresh cilantro leaves.
1 tablespoon of lemon juice.
2 tablespoons olive oil.
1 clove garlic, minced
A pinch of salt and pepper.

Instructions:

Cook quinoa or brown rice according per the package directions.

Roast sweet potato cubes on a baking sheet at 400°F for 20 minutes, or until soft.

While the base cooks, make the dressing. Blend all dressing ingredients in a food processor until smooth.

Fill the bowls with cooked base, spinach/kale, roasted sweet potato, cherry tomatoes, avocado, feta cheese, sunflower seeds, and seasonings.

Drizzle with green goddess dressing and enjoy!

2. Detoxing Avocado Toast with Spicy Radish Top Pesto

Ingredients:

1 slice of toasted whole wheat bread.

1/2 avocado, mashed

1/4 cup of radish top pesto (see recipe below for pesto procedures)

1/4 cup of microgreens.

Sprinkle of hemp seeds

A pinch of red pepper flakes (optional)

Radish Top Pesto

1 cup radish tops, roughly chopped.

1/4 cup raw cashews.

1 clove garlic.
1 tablespoon of olive oil.
1/4 cup shredded Parmesan cheese (optional)
Add salt and pepper to taste.

Instructions:
To make the pesto, combine all of the ingredients in a food processor and blend until smooth. Adjust the seasoning with salt and pepper.
Spread mashed avocado on bread. Optional toppings include radish top pesto, microgreens, hemp seeds, and red pepper flakes.

3. Anti-inflammatory Chia Seed Porridge:
Ingredients:
1/2 cup chia seeds.
1 cup almond milk (or other plant-based milk)
1/4 cup frozen berries.
1/4 cup chopped fresh mango.
1/4 teaspoon of ground turmeric.
A pinch of cinnamon
A handful of sliced almonds.
Add honey or maple syrup to taste.

Instructions:

In a jar or bowl, blend the chia seeds and milk. Stir thoroughly and set aside for at least 15 minutes, or overnight for thicker porridge.

Garnish with frozen berries, mango, turmeric, cinnamon, and almonds.

Drizzle with honey or maple syrup to add sweetness (optional).

4. Immune Boosting Berry Bliss Bowls:

Ingredients:

1 cup Greek or coconut yoghurt

1/2 cup mixed berries, fresh or frozen.

1/4 cup granola.

1/4 cup chopped banana.

1 tablespoon of chia seeds.

1/2 teaspoon of hemp seeds.

Optional: drizzle with honey or maple syrup.

Instructions:

In a bowl, combine yoghurt, berries, granola, banana, chia seeds, and hemp seeds.

To add sweetness, drizzle with honey or maple syrup (optional).

5. Turmeric Latte With Ginger And Collagen:
Ingredients:
1 cup unsweetened almond milk (or other plant-based milk)
1/2 teaspoon of ground turmeric.
1/4 teaspoon of ground ginger.
1 scoop of collagen peptides (optional).
1/4 teaspoon of vanilla extract.
A pinch of black pepper.
Add honey or maple syrup to taste.

Instructions:
In a small saucepan, heat the milk over medium heat.
Mix in the turmeric, ginger, collagen (if using), vanilla extract, and black pepper.
Heat until heated through, but do not boil.
Pour into a mug and top with honey or maple syrup, if desired.

6. Lemon Tahini Energy Balls.
Ingredients:
1 cup of pitted Medjool dates
1/2 cup rolled oats.
1/4 cup unsweetened tahini.
2 teaspoons of lemon juice.
1 tablespoon of chia seeds.
1/4 teaspoon of ground cinnamon.

A pinch of sea salt.
Optional: coconut flakes for rolling (approximately 1/4 cup).

Instructions:
Combine all ingredients except the coconut flakes (if using) in a food processor.
Process until sticky and thoroughly blended, scraping down the sides as needed.
If the mixture is too dry, add a tablespoon of water at a time until it comes together smoothly.
Roll the mixture into bite-sized balls using your hands.
Roll each ball in coconut flakes to coat.
Refrigerate in an airtight container for up to one week.

7. Almond Butter Banana Muesli Cups.
Ingredients:
1 cup rolled oats.
1/2 cup of unsweetened almond butter.
1/4 cup mashed banana.
1/4 cup honey.
1/4 cup milk of choice.
1/4 teaspoon of ground cinnamon.
A pinch of sea salt.

Optional toppings include chopped nuts, seeds, or dried fruit.

Instructions:

Preheat the oven to 350°F (175°C). Grease a muffin tray or use cupcake liners.

In a large mixing bowl, add oats, almond butter, mashed banana, honey, milk, cinnamon, and salt.

Mix thoroughly until a thick batter develops.

Divide the batter evenly into the muffin tray cups.

Bake for 15 to 20 minutes, or until golden brown and set.

Allow it cool somewhat before topping with the preferred seasonings (optional).

Refrigerate in an airtight container for up to three days.

8. Blueberry Acai Overnight Oats.

Ingredients:

1/2 cup rolled oats.

1/2 cup of unsweetened plant-based milk.

1/4 cup of unsweetened acai puree.

1/4 cup frozen blueberries.

1/4 cup Greek yoghurt (optional).

1 tablespoon of chia seeds.

One tablespoon honey (optional)

1/4 teaspoon of ground cinnamon.

A pinch of sea salt.
Optional toppings include fresh or frozen berries, granola, or chopped almonds.

Instructions:
In a jar or container, combine the oats, milk, acai puree, blueberries, yoghurt (if using), chia seeds, honey (if using), cinnamon, and salt.
Stir thoroughly and cover securely.
Refrigerate overnight or at least four hours.
In the morning, whisk again and top with your preferred additions.

9. Sweet Potato hash with kale and poached eggs.

Ingredients:
One medium sweet potato, peeled and chopped
1 tablespoon of olive oil.
1/2 onion, chopped.
1 clove garlic, minced
1 cup kale, chopped
1/4 cup crumbled feta cheese (optional).
2 eggs
1 tablespoon vinegar.
Add salt and pepper to taste.
Optional toppings include avocado slices, spicy sauce, and fresh herbs.

Instructions:

In a large skillet, heat olive oil over medium heat. Cook sweet potatoes for 5-7 minutes, or until they begin to soften.

Add the onion and garlic and simmer for another 3-4 minutes, or until softened.

Stir in the kale and simmer until wilted.

Season with salt and pepper to taste.

In a separate small saucepan, bring water and vinegar to a simmer. Break each egg into a small basin.

Gently swirl the water to form a vortex, then delicately slide each egg into the water. Poach for 3-4 minutes, or until desired level of doneness.

Serve sweet potato hash topped with eggs, feta cheese (if using), and any additional toppings.

10. Apple Cinnamon Quinoa Bowl

Ingredients:

1/2 cup of cooked quinoa.

1/2 apple, diced.

1/4 cup of unsweetened almond milk.

1 tablespoon of chia seeds.

Half a teaspoon of crushed cinnamon

1/4 teaspoon of ground ginger.

A pinch of sea salt.

Optional toppings include chopped nuts, seeds, dried fruit, and a drizzle of honey.

Instructions:
If you don't have any cooked quinoa on hand, cook 1/2 cup using your chosen technique. It is recommended that you rinse before cooking.
In a bowl, combine the cooked quinoa with 1/2 diced apple, 1/4 cup unsweetened almond milk, 1 tablespoon chia seeds, 1/2 teaspoon ground cinnamon, 1/4 teaspoon ground ginger, and a dash of sea salt.
Cover the bowl and chill for at least 15 minutes, or overnight for a thicker texture. This allows the flavors to come together and the chia seeds to absorb moisture.
Stir the mixture again, then top with your favorite ingredients. Some options include chopped nuts (walnuts, pecans, almonds), seeds (chia, sunflower, pumpkin), dried fruit (cranberries, raisins, dates), honey, or a dollop of yoghurt.

Lymph Boosting Smoothies

1. The Ultimate Immune Smoothie:
Ingredients:
1 cup leafy greens (spinach, kale, or a combination)
1/2 cup mixed berries (blueberries or raspberries)
1/2 orange, peeled and segmented
1/2 banana, frozen
1 inch ginger root, peeled and sliced
1/2 cup plain yoghurt, Greek or dairy-free.
1 tablespoon of chia seeds.
1 cup unsweetened plant-based milk or water.
Optional: One scoop of plant-based protein powder.

Instructions:
Add all of the ingredients to your blender.
Blend until smooth and creamy.
Enjoy right away!

2. Beetroot and Berry Blend:
Ingredients:
One small beetroot, boiled and chopped
1/2 cup mixed berries.
1/2 apple, cored and cut.
1/2 banana, frozen
1 cup plant-based milk, unsweetened
1/2 teaspoon of lemon juice.

1/4 teaspoon of ground ginger.
A pinch of sea salt.

Instructions:
Add all of the ingredients to your blender.
Blend until smooth and creamy.
Optional: Strain over a fine-mesh sieve to achieve a smoother texture.
Enjoy right away!

3. Citrus Cleansing Smoothie:
Ingredients:
One grapefruit, peeled and segmented
One orange, peeled and segmented
1/2 lemon, peeled and squeezed.
1/2 cup pineapple chunks, frozen
1/2 cucumber, peeled and sliced.
1 cup unsweetened plant-based milk or water.
1/2 teaspoon of grated ginger.
A pinch of cayenne pepper (optional).

Instructions:
Add all of the ingredients to your blender.
Blend until smooth and creamy.
Enjoy right away!

4. Superfood Green Smoothie:

Ingredients:

1 bunch of baby spinach.

1 bunch kale with stems removed

1/2 avocado, peeled and pitted.

1/2 banana, frozen

1/2 cup pineapple chunks, frozen

1 tablespoon of chia seeds.

1 cup of unsweetened plant-based milk.

1 scoop of green superfood powder (optional).

1/2 teaspoon spirulina powder (optional).

Instructions:

Add all of the ingredients to your blender.

Blend until smooth and creamy.

Enjoy right away!

5. Purple Powerhouse Smoothie.

Ingredients:

1/2 cup blueberries.

1/2 cup raspberries.

1/4 cup blackberries.

1/2 beetroot, boiled and diced.

1/2 banana, frozen

1 tablespoon of acai powder.

1 cup plant-based milk, unsweetened

1/2 teaspoon of vanilla extract.

A pinch of ground cinnamon.

Instructions:
Add all of the ingredients to your blender.
Blend until smooth and creamy.
Enjoy right away!

6. Pineapple Paradise Smoothie.

Ingredients:
1 cup of frozen pineapple pieces.
1/2 cup of frozen mango chunks.
1/2 cup baby spinach.
1/4 cup unsweetened coconut milk.
1/4 cup plain yoghurt, Greek or ordinary.
One tablespoon honey (optional)
1/2 teaspoon of ground ginger.
A pinch of turmeric (optional).
Ice cubes (Optional)

Instructions:
Blend all of the ingredients until smooth and creamy.
Add more coconut milk or ice cubes as needed to achieve the desired consistency.
Pour into glasses, and enjoy!

7. Matcha Magic Smoothie.

Ingredients:

1/2 cup of frozen banana pieces.

1/4 cup rolled oats.

1/2 cup of unsweetened almond milk.

1/2 cup spinach.

1 scoop of matcha powder.

Half a teaspoon of crushed cinnamon

1/4 teaspoon of ground ginger.

A pinch of sea salt.

Ice cubes (Optional)

Instructions:

Blend all of the ingredients until smooth and creamy. Add more almond milk or ice cubes as needed to achieve the desired consistency.

Pour into glasses, and enjoy!

8. Spiced carrot and ginger smoothie:

Ingredients:

One medium carrot, peeled and sliced

1/2 cup of frozen mango chunks.

1/4 cup unsweetened plant-based milk.

1/4 cup plain yoghurt, Greek or ordinary.

1 tablespoon of chia seeds.

1/2 teaspoon of ground ginger.

1/4 teaspoon of ground turmeric.

A pinch of ground cinnamon.
A pinch of black pepper.
Ice cubes (Optional)

Instructions:
Blend all of the ingredients until smooth and creamy.
If necessary, add more milk or ice cubes to achieve
the desired consistency.
Pour into glasses, and enjoy!

9. Tropical Green Smoothie:
Ingredients:
1 cup of frozen pineapple pieces.
1/2 cup of frozen mango chunks.
1/2 cup baby spinach.
1/4 cup unsweetened coconut water.
1/4 cup plain yoghurt, Greek or ordinary.
1 tablespoon of chia seeds.
1/2 teaspoon of ground ginger.
A pinch of turmeric (optional).
Ice cubes (Optional)

Instructions:
Blend all of the ingredients until smooth and creamy.
To adjust the consistency, add more coconut water or
ice cubes as needed.
Pour into glasses, and enjoy!

10. Cherry Bomb Smoothie:

Ingredients:

1 cup frozen cherries.

1/2 cup of frozen banana pieces.

1/4 cup of unsweetened almond milk.

1/4 cup plain yoghurt, Greek or ordinary.

One tablespoon honey (optional)

Half a teaspoon of crushed cinnamon

A pinch of ground nutmeg.

Ice cubes (Optional)

Instructions:

Blend all of the ingredients until smooth and creamy.

Add more almond milk or ice cubes as needed to achieve the desired consistency.

Pour into glasses, and enjoy!

Nutrition-Packed Muffins and Scones

1. Gluten-free Zucchini Muffins.
Ingredients:
1 cup almond flour.
1/4 cup coconut flour.
1/2 teaspoon of baking powder.
1/4 teaspoon of baking soda.
1/4 teaspoon of ground cinnamon.
1/4 teaspoon ground nutmeg.
Pinch of salt.
One huge egg.
1/4 cup honey.
1/4 cup unsweetened applesauce.
1/4 cup melted coconut oil.
1/2 cup shredded zucchini.
1/2 cup chopped walnuts.

Instructions:
Preheat the oven to 375° Fahrenheit (190° Celsius).
Line the muffin tray with paper liners.
In a large basin, combine almond flour, coconut flour, baking powder, baking soda, cinnamon, nutmeg, and salt.
In a separate bowl, whisk together the egg, honey, applesauce, and coconut oil.

Mix the wet ingredients into the dry ingredients until just mixed. Don't overmix.
Fold in the grated zucchini and chopped walnuts.
Divide the batter evenly among the prepared muffin cups.
Bake for 20 to 25 minutes, or until a toothpick inserted in the centre comes out clean.
Let cool in the pan for 5 minutes before transferring to a wire rack to finish cooling.

Tips:
To make a moister muffin, add 1/4 cup mashed banana or unsweetened applesauce.
You can use any other chopped nuts instead of walnuts.
For an added crunch, sprinkle the muffin tops with chopped nuts or cinnamon before baking.

2. Flaxseed and Cranberry Muffins

Ingredients:
1 cup rolled oats.
1/4 cup ground flaxseed.
1/2 teaspoon of baking powder.
1/4 teaspoon of baking soda.
1/4 teaspoon of ground cinnamon.
Pinch of salt.
One huge egg.

1/4 cup honey.

1/4 cup unsweetened applesauce.

1/4 cup milk of choice.

1/2 cup dried cranberries.

1/4 cup of chopped walnuts (optional).

Instructions:

Preheat the oven to 375° Fahrenheit (190° Celsius).

Line the muffin tray with paper liners.

In a blender or food processor, crush the rolled oats until they are the consistency of flour.

In a large mixing bowl, combine oat flour, ground flaxseed, baking powder, baking soda, cinnamon, and salt.

In a separate bowl, whisk together the egg, honey, applesauce, and milk.

Mix the wet ingredients into the dry ingredients until just mixed. Don't overmix.

Fold in the dried cranberries and chopped walnuts (if using).

Divide the batter evenly among the prepared muffin cups.

Bake for 20 to 25 minutes, or until a toothpick inserted in the center comes out clean.

Let cool in the pan for 5 minutes before transferring to a wire rack to finish cooling.

Tips:

If you like, you can use chia seeds instead of ground flaxseed.

To make the muffins sweeter, add a spoonful of brown sugar to the wet ingredients.

You can use any dried fruit you like, including raisins, cherries, and chopped dates.

3. Spinach and Feta Scones

Ingredients:

2 cups all-purpose flour.

1 tablespoon of baking powder.

1/2 teaspoon of baking soda.

1/2 teaspoon of salt.

1/4 cup cold, unsalted butter, cubed

1/2 cup packed fresh spinach, chopped.

1/2 cup crumbled feta cheese.

1 cup buttermilk (or 1 cup milk and 1 tablespoon lemon juice)

One egg yolk, beaten

Instructions:

Preheat the oven to 425° Fahrenheit (220° Celsius). Line a baking sheet with parchment paper.

In a large mixing basin, combine flour, baking powder, baking soda, and salt.

Using a pastry cutter or fork, combine the chilled butter and dry ingredients until the mixture resembles coarse crumbs.

Combine the chopped spinach and crumbled feta cheese.

Add the buttermilk (or milk mixture) and egg yolk to the dry ingredients and mix until a dough forms. Don't overmix.

Turn the dough out onto a lightly floured board and shape it into a 1-inch-thick circle.

Use a knife or cookie cutter to cut the dough into 8-12 wedges. Place the scones on the prepared baking sheet, leaving some space between them.

Brush the scones' tops with milk or egg wash (optional).

Bake for 15-20 minutes, until golden brown and well done.

Allow it cool on the baking pan for a few minutes before serving.

Tips:

You can use kale or Swiss chard instead of spinach.

If you prefer vegan scones, skip the cheese.

Serve the scones warm, with butter, jam, or honey.

4. Blueberries with Chia Seed Muffins

Ingredients:

1 1/2 cups all-purpose flour.

1/2 cup granulated sugar.

2 tablespoons baking powder.

1/2 teaspoon of baking soda.

1/4 teaspoon salt.

1/4 cup chia seeds.

One huge egg.

1/4 cup milk.

1/4 cup vegetable oil.

1 teaspoon of vanilla extract.

1 cup blueberries, fresh or frozen.

Instructions:

Preheat the oven to 400° F (200° C). Line the muffin tray with paper liners.

In a large mixing basin, combine flour, sugar, baking powder, baking soda, and salt.

Stir in the chia seeds.

In a separate bowl, whisk together the egg, milk, oil, and vanilla extract.

Stir the wet and dry ingredients together until just mixed. Don't overmix.

Gently fold in the blueberries.

Divide the batter evenly among the prepared muffin cups.

Bake for 20 to 25 minutes, or until a toothpick inserted in the centre comes out clean.
Let cool in the pan for 5 minutes before transferring to a wire rack to finish cooling.

Tips:
You can use raspberries or strawberries instead of blueberries.
To make a streusel topping, combine 1/4 cup flour, 1/4 cup brown sugar, and 2 tablespoons cubed cold butter; crumble on top of the batter before baking.
To make a vegan muffin, substitute ground flaxseed or chia seeds for the eggs.

5. Sweet Potato and Raisin Muffins.
Ingredients:
1 cup mashed sweet potato (about one medium sweet potato)
1/2 cup all-purpose flour.
1/2 cup of whole wheat flour.
1/2 cup brown sugar.
2 tablespoons baking powder.
1 teaspoon of cinnamon.
1/2 teaspoon nutmeg.
1/4 teaspoon salt.
One huge egg.
1/4 cup milk.

1/4 cup melted butter.
1/2 cup raisins.

Instructions:
Preheat the oven to 400° F (200° C). Line the muffin tray with paper liners.
In a large mixing basin, combine the mashed sweet potatoes, flours, brown sugar, baking powder, cinnamon, nutmeg, and salt.
In a separate bowl, whisk together the egg, milk, and melted butter.
Stir the wet and dry ingredients together until just mixed. Don't overmix.
Gently fold in the raisins.
Divide the batter evenly among the prepared muffin cups.
Bake for 20 to 25 minutes, or until a toothpick inserted in the centre comes out clean.
Let cool in the pan for 5 minutes before transferring to a wire rack to finish cooling.

Tips:
If you don't like raisins, you can use alternative chopped nuts.
To make a streusel topping, combine 1/4 cup flour, 1/4 cup brown sugar, and 2 tablespoons cubed cold

butter, then sprinkle on top of the batter before baking.
You can substitute almond milk or another plant-based milk for dairy milk.

6. Carrots and Ginger Muffins:

Ingredients:
1 cup grated carrots (about two medium carrots)
1 1/2 cups all-purpose flour.
1/2 cup granulated sugar.
2 tablespoons baking powder.
1 teaspoon of baking soda.
1/2 teaspoon of ground ginger.
1/4 teaspoon cinnamon.
1/4 teaspoon salt.
One huge egg.
1/4 cup milk.
1/4 cup vegetable oil.
1 teaspoon of vanilla extract.
1/2 cup of chopped walnuts (optional)

Instructions:
Preheat the oven to 400° F (200° C). Line the muffin tray with paper liners.
In a large mixing basin, combine flour, sugar, baking powder, soda, ginger, cinnamon, and salt.
Stir in the grated carrots.

In a separate bowl, whisk together the egg, milk, oil, and vanilla extract.

Stir the wet and dry ingredients together until just mixed. Don't overmix.

Mix in the chopped walnuts (if using).

Divide the batter evenly among the prepared muffin cups.

Bake for 20 to 25 minutes, or until a toothpick inserted in the centre comes out clean.

Let cool in the pan for 5 minutes before transferring to a wire rack to finish cooling.

Tips:

Instead of walnuts, you can use other chopped nuts or dried fruit.

To make a streusel topping, combine 1/4 cup flour, 1/4 cup brown sugar, and 2 tablespoons cubed cold butter; crumble on top of the batter before baking.

To make a vegan muffin, substitute chia seeds or ground flaxseed for the eggs.

7. Pumpkin Spice Muffins:

Ingredients:

1 cup of canned pumpkin puree.

1 1/2 cups all-purpose flour.

1/2 cup granulated sugar.

2 tablespoons baking powder.

1 teaspoon of baking soda
1 teaspoon ground cinnamon.
1/2 teaspoon of ground ginger.
1/4 teaspoon ground nutmeg.
1/4 teaspoon salt.
One huge egg.
1/4 cup milk.
1/4 cup vegetable oil.
1 teaspoon of vanilla extract.
1/2 cup of chopped pecans (optional)

Instructions:
Preheat the oven to 400° F (200° C). Line the muffin tray with paper liners.
In a large basin, combine the flour, sugar, baking powder, baking soda, cinnamon, ginger, nutmeg, and salt.
Stir in the pumpkin puree.
In a separate bowl, whisk together the egg, milk, oil, and vanilla extract.
Stir the wet and dry ingredients together until just mixed. Don't overmix.
Fold in the chopped pecans (optional). Divide the batter evenly among the prepared muffin cups.
Bake for 20 to 25 minutes, or until a toothpick inserted in the centre comes out clean.

Let cool in the pan for 5 minutes before transferring to a wire rack to finish cooling.

Tips:
Instead of pecans, you can use other chopped nuts or dried fruit.

To make a streusel topping, combine 1/4 cup flour, 1/4 cup brown sugar, 2 tablespoons cubed cold butter, and 1/2 teaspoon cinnamon. Crumble over the batter before baking.

To make a vegan muffin, substitute chia seeds or ground flaxseed for the eggs.

8. Whole Wheat Banana Nut Muffins

Ingredients:

1 1/2 cups whole wheat flour.

1/2 cup granulated sugar.

2 tablespoons baking powder.

1 teaspoon of baking soda.

1/2 teaspoon of salt.

1/2 cup mashed ripe bananas (about two bananas)

1/4 cup milk.

1/4 cup vegetable oil.

One huge egg.

1/2 cup chopped walnuts.

Instructions:
Preheat the oven to 400° F (200° C). Line the muffin tray with paper liners.
In a large mixing basin, combine flour, sugar, baking powder, baking soda, and salt.
In a separate bowl, mash the bananas. Whisk the milk, oil, and egg into the mashed bananas until thoroughly incorporated.
Stir the wet and dry ingredients together until just mixed. Don't overmix.
Fold in the chopped walnuts.
Divide the batter evenly among the prepared muffin cups.
Bake for 20 to 25 minutes, or until a toothpick inserted in the centre comes out clean.
Let cool in the pan for 5 minutes before transferring to a wire rack to finish cooling.

Tips:
Instead of walnuts, you can use other chopped nuts or dried fruit.
To make a streusel topping, combine 1/4 cup flour, 1/4 cup brown sugar, and 2 tablespoons cubed cold butter, then sprinkle on top of the batter before baking.
You can substitute almond milk or any plant-based milk for dairy milk.

9. Lemon Poppyseed Muffins:

Ingredients:

1 1/2 cups all-purpose flour.

1/2 cup granulated sugar.

2 tablespoons baking powder.

1/2 teaspoon of salt.

1/4 cup poppy seeds.

1/4 cup grated lemon zest (about one lemon)

One huge egg.

1/4 cup milk.

1/4 cup vegetable oil.

1 tablespoon of lemon juice.

1/4 cup powdered sugar (optional; glaze)

1 tablespoon milk (optional for glazing)

Instructions:

Preheat the oven to 400° F (200° C). Line the muffin tray with paper liners.

In a large bowl, combine the flour, sugar, baking powder, salt, and poppy seeds.

Stir in the lemon zest.

In a separate bowl, whisk together the egg, milk, oil, and lemon juice.

Stir the wet and dry ingredients together until just mixed. Don't overmix.

Divide the batter evenly among the prepared muffin cups.

Bake for 20 to 25 minutes, or until a toothpick inserted in the centre comes out clean.

Let cool in the pan for 5 minutes before transferring to a wire rack to finish cooling.

For an optional glaze, combine powdered sugar and milk until smooth. Drizzle over the cooled muffins.

Tips:

If you prefer not to use the glaze, you can do so.

You can substitute almond milk or any plant-based milk for dairy milk.

10. Apple cinnamon scones:

Ingredients:

2 cups all-purpose flour.

1/4 cup granulated sugar.

2 tablespoons baking powder.

1/2 teaspoon of baking soda.

Half a teaspoon of crushed cinnamon

1/4 teaspoon salt.

1/2 cup cold, unsalted butter, cubed

1/2 cup chopped apples

1/4 cup milk.

One huge egg yolk.

1 tablespoon milk (to brush)

1 tablespoon granulated sugar (to sprinkle)

Instructions:

Preheat the oven to 425° Fahrenheit (220° Celsius).

Line a baking sheet with parchment paper.

In a large mixing basin, combine flour, sugar, baking powder, baking soda, cinnamon, and salt.

Using a pastry cutter or fork, combine the chilled butter and dry ingredients until the mixture resembles coarse crumbs.

Mix in the chopped apple.

In a separate bowl, mix together the milk and egg yolk.

Combine the wet and dry ingredients and whisk just until a dough forms. Don't overmix.

Turn the dough out onto a lightly floured board and shape it into a 1-inch-thick circle.

Use a knife or cookie cutter to cut the dough into 8-12 wedges. Place the scones on the prepared baking sheet, leaving some space between them.

Brush the tops of the scones with milk.

Sprinkle with granulated sugar.

Bake for 15-20 minutes, until golden brown and well done.

Allow it cool on the baking pan for a few minutes before serving.

Tips:

Berries, peaches, and pears can be used instead of apples.

Brown sugar, rather than granulated sugar, has a deeper flavor.

You can leave out the egg yolk and brush the scones with melted butter before baking.

Serve the scones warm, with butter, jam, or honey.

Healthy Snacks

1. Roasted Chickpea & Herb Snack Mix:
Ingredients:
1 can (15 oz) of chickpeas, drained and rinsed
1 tablespoon of olive oil.
1 teaspoon of dried oregano.
1/2 teaspoon of smoked paprika.
1/4 teaspoon of garlic powder.
1/4 teaspoon salt.
1/4 teaspoon of black pepper.
1/4 cup chopped fresh herbs (parsley, rosemary, or thyme)
Optional ingredients include shredded cheese, chopped nuts, dried fruit, and spices such as cumin or chilli powder.

Instructions:
Preheat the oven to 400° F (200° C). Line a baking sheet with parchment paper.
Dry the chickpeas with a paper towel.
In a bowl, combine the chickpeas, olive oil, oregano, paprika, garlic powder, salt, and pepper.
Spread the chickpeas evenly on the prepared baking sheet.
Roast for 20-25 minutes, until golden brown and crispy, tossing periodically.

Allow it cool somewhat before adding the fresh herbs and other preferred toppings.

Tips:
For a hotter snack, add a sprinkle of cayenne pepper to the seasoning mixture.
You can customise the spices by adding curry powder, turmeric, or nutritional yeast.
This snack combination is best consumed within a few days.

2. Homemade Granola Bites:
Ingredients:
1 cup rolled oats.
1/2 cup chopped nuts (such as almonds, pecans, or walnuts)
1/4 cup dried fruit (such as raisins, cranberries, or chopped dates)
1/4 cup shredded coconut
1/4 cup honey or maple syrup.
1 tablespoon of heated coconut oil.
1/4 teaspoon of ground cinnamon.
1/8 teaspoon of ground ginger.
Pinch of salt.

Instructions:
Preheat the oven to 350°F (175°C). Line a baking sheet with parchment paper.
In a large bowl, combine the rolled oats, almonds, dried fruit, and coconut.
In a separate bowl, combine the honey or maple syrup, coconut oil, cinnamon, ginger, and salt.
Stir the wet and dry ingredients together until thoroughly blended.
Place tablespoons of the mixture on the prepared baking sheet.
Bake for 15 to 20 minutes, or until golden brown and somewhat hard.
Allow to cool completely on the baking pan.

Tips:
You can substitute chia seeds or flaxseeds for some of the oats.
Add a teaspoon of nut butter to the wet ingredients for added flavor and protein.
Store leftover granola bites in an airtight container in the refrigerator for up to a week.

3. Raw vegetable sticks with hummus or guacamole:

Ingredients:

Choose your favourite vegetables, such as carrots, celery, cucumbers, bell peppers, broccoli florets, and cherry tomatoes.

Hummus or Guacamole

Optional extras include pita bread, crackers, and sliced apple or pear.

Instructions:

Wash and prepare your desired vegetables. Cut them into sticks or bite-size chunks.

Serve the vegetables alongside hummus or guacamole for dipping.

Serve with pita bread, crackers, or sliced fruit for a more filling snack.

Tips:

Include both softer and crunchier vegetables to give your dish a diversity of textures.

Try different flavors of hummus or guacamole.

To add flavor, sprinkle the vegetables with spices such as paprika or za'atar.

4. Fresh Fruit Salad With Honey Yoghurt Dressing

Ingredients:

2 cups mixed seasonal fruits (such as berries, melon, grapes, apple, and mango)

1/4 cup plain yoghurt, Greek or ordinary.

1 tablespoon honey.

1/2 teaspoon of lemon juice.

A pinch of cinnamon (optional).

Fresh mint leaves for garnish (optional).

Instructions:

Wash and cut your desired fruits into bite-sized pieces.

In a small bowl, combine the yoghurt, honey, lemon juice, and cinnamon (if using).

Toss the fruit salad in the dressing until it is evenly coated.

Garnish with fresh mint leaves (optional), and serve chilled.

Tips:

Adjust the amount of honey to match the sweetness of your fruits.

Other items you can add to the dressing include vanilla flavour, ginger, and chopped almonds.

To make the dressing thicker, use less yoghurt or add a tablespoon of chia seeds.

5. Dark chocolate-covered frozen bananas:
Ingredients:
Two ripe bananas, peeled and sliced
1/2 cup dark chocolate chips.
Optional toppings include chopped nuts, shredded coconut, and sprinkles.

Instructions:
Line a baking sheet with parchment paper.
Place the banana slices on the prepared baking sheet and freeze for at least two hours, or until solid.
Melt the chocolate chips in a microwave-safe bowl in short bursts while stirring, or in a double boiler.
Dip the frozen banana slices into the melted chocolate and coat them evenly.
Return the covered bananas to the baking sheet and add any desired toppings.
Freeze for a further 30 minutes, or until the chocolate has set. Enjoy!

Tips:
Dip the bananas in chocolate using a fork or a toothpick.

While the chocolate is melting, add a teaspoon of coconut oil to make a thinner coating.

You can use many varieties of chocolate, including milk chocolate and white chocolate.

6. Roasted edamame

Ingredients:

1 cup frozen, shelled edamame

1 tablespoon of olive oil.

1/2 teaspoon of sea salt.

Optional additions include garlic powder, black pepper, and chilli flakes.

Instructions:

Preheat the oven to 400° F (200° C).

Line a baking sheet with parchment paper.

Place the frozen edamame in a single layer on the prepared baking sheet.

Drizzle with olive oil and season with salt and any desired ingredients.

Roast for 15-20 minutes, or until edamame is soft and gently browned.

Allow to cool slightly before serving.

Tips:
Edamame can be cooked in the microwave rather than the oven. Follow the directions on the packaging.
To make the seasonings hotter, add a sprinkle of cayenne pepper.
You can also cook edamame in an air fryer at 400°F for 10-12 minutes.

7. Hardboiled eggs with spices
Ingredients:
4 eggs
One tablespoon vinegar (white or apple cider)
1 teaspoon salt.
Optional spices include black peppercorns, bay leaves, and chilli flakes.

Instructions:
Place the eggs in a saucepan in a single layer.
Cover the eggs with cold water, then add the vinegar and salt.
Bring the water to a boil on high heat.
Once boiling, remove the pan from the heat and cover tightly.
Allow the eggs to sit in the hot water for 10-12 minutes for soft-boiled eggs and 15-17 minutes for hard-boiled eggs.

Drain the hot water and run cold water over the eggs until they're cool enough to touch.
Peel the eggs and enjoy!

Tips:
Before placing the eggs in the water, break them slightly to make peeling simpler.
For added flavour, try adding black peppercorns, bay leaves, or chilli flakes to the water.
Hard-boiled eggs can be stored in the refrigerator for up to one week.

8. Rice Cake topped with avocado and tomatoes

Ingredients:
Two rice cakes.
1/2 avocado, thinly sliced.
One tomato, thinly sliced
A pinch of salt and pepper (optional)
Additional toppings (optional): chopped herbs (cilantro, basil), lemon juice, hot sauce, and Everything Bagel spice.

Instructions:
If desired, softly toast the rice cakes in the toaster or oven.

Spread the avocado evenly on one rice cake after lightly mashing it with a fork.
Arrange the tomato slices on top of the avocado.
Season to taste with salt and pepper, and if preferred, add lemon juice or spicy sauce.
Sprinkle with additional toppings as desired.

9. Roasted vegetables with garlic aioli:

Ingredients:
2 cups chopped veggies (e.g., broccoli, cauliflower, carrots, zucchini)
1 tablespoon of olive oil.
1/2 teaspoon of dried oregano.
1/4 teaspoon of garlic powder.
A pinch of salt and pepper.
For the garlic aioli:
1/2 cup mayonnaise.
1 clove garlic, minced
1/4 teaspoon of lemon juice.
Pinch of salt.

Instructions:
Preheat the oven to 400° F (200° C). Line a baking sheet with parchment paper.
Mix the vegetables with olive oil, oregano, garlic powder, salt, and pepper.

Spread the vegetables evenly on the prepared baking sheet.

Roast for 20 to 25 minutes, or until soft and gently browned.

While the vegetables roast, make the aioli:

In a small bowl, combine mayonnaise, garlic, lemon juice, and salt.

Serve the roasted vegetables beside the garlic aioli for dipping.

Tips:

You can make this dish with any mix of your favorite vegetables.

To make vegan aioli, use vegan mayonnaise or similar plant-based spread.

If preferred, drizzle the veggies with balsamic vinegar or another dressing prior to serving.

10. Air-fried sweet potato wedges:

Ingredients:

one sweet potato, cleaned and cut into wedges

1 tablespoon of olive oil.

1/2 teaspoon paprika.

1/4 teaspoon of garlic powder.

A pinch of salt and pepper.

Instructions:
Preheat your air fryer to 400 °F (200°C).
In a mixing dish, combine the sweet potato wedges with the olive oil, paprika, garlic powder, salt, and pepper.
Arrange the wedges in a single layer in the air fryer basket, making sure they do not overlap.
Air fried for 15-20 minutes, or until tender and golden brown. Flip halfway through.
Serve immediately with your preferred dipping sauce, such as ketchup, barbecue sauce, or ranch dressing.

Tips:
To get crispier wedges, soak the sweet potatoes in cold water for 15 minutes before cutting and air-frying.
To change the flavor, apply spices such as cumin, cayenne pepper, or chilli powder.
If you don't have an air fryer, bake the sweet potato wedges in a preheated oven at 400°F (200°C) for 25-30 minutes, flipping once halfway through.

Guilt-free Cookies and Bars

1. Almond Butter Protein Bites:
Ingredients:
1/2 cup of unsweetened almond butter.
1/4 cup rolled oats.
1/4 cup of pitted Medjool dates, chopped
2 tablespoons chia seeds.
1 tablespoon protein powder (chocolate or vanilla)
A pinch of sea salt.
Optional: Extra chopped nuts, shredded coconut, or dried fruit.

Instructions:
In a medium mixing dish, add almond butter, oats, dates, chia seeds, protein powder, and salt.
Mix thoroughly until a sticky dough forms. If the mixture is too dry, add a tablespoon of water or unsweetened almond milk at a time until it comes together smoothly.
Using your hands, roll the dough into balls approximately one inch in diameter.
Arrange the bites on a baking sheet lined with parchment paper.
Refrigerate for at least 30 minutes, or until firm.
Refrigerate in an airtight container for up to one week.

2. No-bake Peanut Butter and Oat Bites:

Ingredients:

1/2 cup of unsweetened peanut butter.

1/4 cup honey.

1/2 cup rolled oats.

1/4 cup flaxseed meal.

1/4 cup chopped dried fruit (such as raisins or cranberries)

Optional: A pinch of cinnamon, crushed coconut, or chopped nuts.

Instructions:

In a large bowl, combine peanut butter and honey. Stir until thoroughly blended and smooth.

Combine rolled oats, flaxseed meal, and dried fruit. Mix thoroughly until everything is evenly incorporated.

Roll the mixture into balls with your hands, aiming for around 1 inch diameter.

Arrange the bites on a baking sheet lined with parchment paper.

Refrigerate for at least 30 minutes, or until firm.

Refrigerate in an airtight container for up to one week.

3. Dark Chocolate and Sea Salt Energy Bites:

Ingredients:

1 cup pitted Medjool dates, chopped

1/2 cup rolled oats.

1/4 cup of unsweetened almond butter.

1/4 cup unsweetened cocoa powder.

1/4 cup chopped dark chocolate (70% or more cacao)

A pinch of sea salt.

Optional: Extra chopped nuts, seeds, or dried fruit.

Instructions:

In a food processor, pulse the Medjool dates until they form a sticky paste.

Combine rolled oats, almond butter, chocolate powder, and salt. Process until everything is well combined and has a dough-like texture.

Stir in the chopped dark chocolate.

Roll the mixture into balls with your hands, aiming for around 1 inch diameter.

Arrange the bites on a baking sheet lined with parchment paper.

Refrigerate for at least 30 minutes, or until firm.

Refrigerate in an airtight container for up to one week.

Tips:

Feel free to adjust the sweetness of these recipes to your liking.

These energy snacks make an excellent grab-and-go snack.

You can change the ingredients according to your dietary needs and preferences.

4. Coconut macaroon bites:

Ingredients:

1 cup unsweetened, shredded coconut

1/3 cup sweetened condensed milk.

1 tablespoon honey.

1/2 teaspoon of vanilla extract.

1/4 teaspoon of almond extract (optional).

Pinch of salt.

Optional: Melted chocolate for dipping (dark, milk, or white)

Instructions:

Preheat the oven to 350°F (175°C). Line a baking sheet with parchment paper.

In a large mixing bowl, add the shredded coconut, condensed milk, honey, vanilla extract, almond extract (if using), and salt. Mix thoroughly until the mixture resembles a sticky dough.

Roll the dough into little balls with your hands or a spoon. Place them on the preheated baking sheet, leaving some space between them.
Bake for 15 to 20 minutes, or until golden brown and somewhat hard.

Allow to cool completely on the baking pan.
To make a chocolate coating, melt your favorite chocolate in a microwave-safe bowl or double boiler. Dip the cooled macaroon bites into the melted chocolate before placing them on a wire rack to set.

Tips:
You can use other extracts instead of almond extract, such as rum or coconut extract.
Bake for fewer minutes if you want a chewier macaron.
To add flavor and texture, roll the macaroon bites in chopped nuts or dried fruit before baking.

5. Pistachio and Date Energy Bites:
Ingredients:
1 cup of pitted Medjool dates
1 cup raw pistachios.
1/4 cup rolled oats.
1/4 cup chia seeds.
2 tablespoons of unsweetened shredded coconut.

2 tablespoons almond butter.
1 tablespoon honey.
1/2 teaspoon cinnamon
Pinch of salt.

Instructions:
In a food processor, pulse the dates and pistachios until roughly chopped.
Add the other ingredients (rolled oats, chia seeds, coconut, almond butter, honey, cinnamon, and salt) and pulse until a sticky dough forms.
Roll the dough into little balls with your hands or a spoon.
Store the energy bites in an airtight container in the refrigerator for up to a week.

Tips:
You can substitute other nuts or seeds for the pistachios, such as almonds, walnuts, or sunflower seeds.
If the mixture is too dry, add a spoonful of water or almond milk at a time until it becomes sticky.
To add flavour and texture, roll the energy bites in additional shredded coconut or cocoa powder.

6. Double Chocolate Chunk Cookies:

Ingredients:

1 cup all-purpose flour.

3/4 cup unsweetened cocoa powder.

1 teaspoon of baking soda.

1/2 teaspoon of salt.

1/2 cup unsalted butter, softened.

1 cup granulated sugar.

1/2 cup packed light brown sugar.

Two large eggs.

1 teaspoon of vanilla extract.

1 cup semisweet chocolate chips.

1/2 cup of chopped dark chocolate (optional)

Instructions:

Preheat the oven to 375° Fahrenheit (190° Celsius).
Line a baking sheet with parchment paper.
In a larger basin, combine the flour, cocoa powder, baking soda, and salt.
In a large mixing bowl, cream together softened butter and sugars until light and fluffy. Beat in the eggs, one at a time, then stir in the vanilla essence.
Gradually add the dry ingredients to the wet ingredients, stirring until just combined. Don't overmix.
Fold in the chocolate chips and the chopped dark chocolate (if using).

Drop heaping spoonful of dough onto the prepared baking sheet, leaving space between each.

Bake for 10 to 12 minutes, or until the edges are firm and the centers are slightly soft.

Allow to cool on the baking sheet for a few minutes before moving to a wire rack to finish cooling.

Tips:

Bake for less minutes if you want chewier cookies.

You can use various nut butters instead of almond butter in the energy bites recipe.

To achieve consistent baking, make sure the cookies are made using room temperature ingredients.

To create a sweet and salty flavour combination, sprinkle sea salt on top of the warm biscuits.

7. Chewy Ginger Molasses Cookies:

Ingredients:

1 1/2 cups all-purpose flour.

1 teaspoon of baking soda.

1/2 teaspoon of salt.

1 teaspoon of ground ginger.

Half a teaspoon of crushed cinnamon

1/4 teaspoon ground cloves.

1/2 cup unsalted butter, softened.

1 cup packed light brown sugar.

1/2 cup granulated sugar.

One huge egg.

1/4 cup unsulphured molasses.

1/4 cup of minced crystallised ginger (optional).

Granulated sugar for rolling is optional.

Instructions:

Preheat the oven to 375° Fahrenheit (190° Celsius).

Line baking pans with parchment paper.

In a larger basin, combine flour, baking soda, salt, and spices.

In a large mixing basin, cream the butter and sugars until light and fluffy. Beat in the egg and molasses until well blended.

Gradually combine the dry and wet ingredients, mixing until just mixed. Fold in the sliced ginger (if using).

Roll the dough into 1-inch balls. Roll the balls in granulated sugar (optional).

Place cookies on prepared baking pans, leaving some space between them.

Bake for 10-12 minutes, or until the edges turn golden brown.

Allow them cool on the baking sheets for a few minutes before transferring to a wire rack to finish cooling.

Tips:
Reduce the baking time for chewier cookies.
You can replace ground ginger with fresh ginger paste (1 tablespoon).
For added flavour, mix with 1/4 cup chopped nuts or dried cranberries.

8. Oatmeal Raisin Cookies.

Ingredients:
1 1/2 cups all-purpose flour.
1 teaspoon of baking soda.
1/2 teaspoon of salt.
1 teaspoon ground cinnamon.
1/2 cup unsalted butter, softened.
3/4 cup packed light brown sugar.
1/2 cup granulated sugar.
One huge egg.
1 teaspoon of vanilla extract.
1 cup rolled oats.
1/2 cup raisins.
1/4 cup of chopped walnuts (optional).

Instructions:
Preheat the oven to 375° Fahrenheit (190° Celsius).
Line baking pans with parchment paper.
In a larger basin, combine flour, baking soda, salt, and cinnamon.

In a large mixing basin, cream the butter and sugars until light and fluffy. Beat in the egg and vanilla essence until incorporated.

Gradually combine the dry and wet ingredients, mixing until just mixed. Fold in the muesli, raisins and walnuts (if using).

Drop dough by the tablespoon onto the prepared baking sheets.

Bake for ten to twelve minutes, or until golden brown.

Allow them cool on the baking sheets for a few minutes before transferring to a wire rack to finish cooling.

Tips:

For a softer cookie, use quick oats, while rolled oats provide a chewier one.

Replace raisins with another dried fruit, such as cranberries, cherries, or dates.

To make a streusel topping, combine 1/4 cup flour, 1/4 cup brown sugar, and 2 tablespoons cubed cold butter, then sprinkle on top of the dough before baking.

9. Chocolate Chip Zucchini Bites:

Ingredients:

1 cup shredded zucchini (packaged)

1/2 cup all-purpose flour.
1/4 cup rolled oats.
1/4 cup unsweetened cocoa powder.
1/4 teaspoon of baking soda.
1/4 teaspoon salt.
1/4 cup melted coconut oil.
1/4 cup honey.
1/4 cup unsweetened applesauce.
One huge egg.
1/2 teaspoon of vanilla extract.
1/2 cup semi-sweet chocolate chips.

Instructions:
Preheat the oven to 350°F (175°C). Line muffin pans with paper liners.
In a larger basin, combine zucchini, flour, oats, cocoa powder, baking soda, and salt.
In a another dish, whisk together coconut oil, honey, applesauce, egg, and vanilla extract.
Add wet ingredients to dry ingredients and mix until just mixed. Fold in chocolate chips.
Divide the batter evenly among the prepared muffin cups.
Bake for 15-20 minutes, or until a toothpick inserted in the center comes out clean.
Let cool in the pan for a few minutes before transferring to a wire rack to cool fully.

Tips:
Before using the shredded zucchini, squeeze it to remove any excess moisture. Instead of chocolate chips, you can use different chopped nuts or dried fruits.

To make a streusel topping, combine 1/4 cup flour, 1/4 cup brown sugar, and 2 tablespoons cubed cold butter, then sprinkle on top of the batter before baking.

These bites can be refrigerated in an airtight container for up to three days.

10. Sunbutter and jelly thumbprint cookies:

Ingredients:

1 1/2 cups all-purpose flour.

1/2 teaspoon of baking soda.

1/4 teaspoon salt.

1/2 cup unsalted butter, softened.

1/2 cup creamy sunflower butter

1/2 cup granulated sugar.

One huge egg.

1/2 cup of your favourite jelly or jam

Instructions:

Preheat the oven to 375° Fahrenheit (190° Celsius).

Line baking pans with parchment paper.

In a larger basin, combine flour, baking soda, and salt.

In a large bowl, mix together butter and sunbutter until light and fluffy. Beat in sugar until blended.

Add the egg and stir until combined.

Gradually combine the dry and wet ingredients, mixing until just mixed.

Roll the dough into 1-inch balls. Place the balls on the prepared baking pans, leaving space between them.

Indent each ball with your thumb or a spoon.

Fill each indentation with roughly 1/2 teaspoon jelly or jam.

Bake for 10-12 minutes, or until the edges turn golden brown.

Allow them cool on the baking sheets for a few minutes before transferring to a wire rack to finish cooling.

Tips:

You can swap sunbutter with peanut butter if you desire.

Use homemade sunbutter or peanut butter to add a deeper flavor.

Before baking, sprinkle sea salt over the cookies to create a sweet and salty flavor combination.

Lymph-Supportive Breads and Wraps

1. Sprouted Grain Sandwich Bread:

Ingredients:

1 cup whole wheat berries

1/2 cup rye berries

1/4 cup spelt berries

1 1/2 cups filtered water

1 tablespoon apple cider vinegar

1 teaspoon salt.

2 tablespoons honey.

2 1/4 cups all-purpose flour

1 tablespoon instant yeast

Instructions:

Sprout the grains: Rinse the whole wheat, rye, and spelt berries in a fine-mesh sieve. Transfer to a large bowl, cover with filtered water, and soak for 8–12 hours. Drain and rinse thoroughly.

Grind the sprouted grains: Using a high-powered blender or grain mill, turn the sprouted grains into coarse flour.

Prepare the dough: In a large mixing bowl, combine the ground sprouted grains, filtered water, apple cider vinegar, and salt. Let it sit for 30 minutes.

Mix in the remaining ingredients: honey, all-purpose flour, and instant yeast. Knead the dough for 10 minutes, either by hand or with a stand mixer, until smooth and elastic.

First rise: Transfer the dough to an oiled basin, cover with plastic wrap, and allow to rise in a warm location for 1-2 hours, or until doubled in size.

Shape and second rise: Punch the dough down and form bread into a loaf. Place in a greased loaf pan, cover with plastic wrap, and allow to rise for a further 30-45 minutes.

Bake: Preheat the oven to 375°F (190°C). Bake the bread for 45 to 50 minutes, or until golden brown and a toothpick inserted in the centre comes out clean.

Cool and enjoy: Allow the bread to cool in the pan for 10 minutes before transferring to a wire rack to finish cooling. Slice, and enjoy!

Tips:

You can replace other berries for the whole wheat, rye, and spelt berries.

If you don't own a high-powered blender or grain mill, you can buy pre-ground sprouted grain flour.

For a sweeter bread, add an extra tablespoon of honey.

2. Gluten-Free Buckwheat Wraps:

Ingredients:

1 cup buckwheat flour

1/2 cup tapioca flour

1/4 cup arrowroot powder

1/2 teaspoon of baking soda.

1/4 teaspoon salt.

1 1/4 cups water

1 tablespoon of olive oil.

Instructions:

In a large bowl, whisk together buckwheat flour, tapioca flour, arrowroot powder, baking soda, and salt.

Add the water and olive oil to the dry ingredients and stir until a thick batter forms.

Heat a lightly greased griddle or frying pan over medium heat. Pour about 1/4 cup of batter onto the pan and swirl to form a thin circle.

Cook for 2-3 minutes per side, or until golden brown and heated through.

Repeat with the remaining batter to form additional wraps.

Fill the wraps with your favorite ingredients, like hummus and veggies, grilled chicken and avocado, or nut butter and berries.

Tips:

You can add 1/4 cup of flaxseed meal to the batter for extra fiber and nutrients.

If the batter is too thick, add a tablespoon of water at a time until it is the right consistency.

You can also cook the wraps in a microwave on high for 30-45 seconds per side.

3. Spelt and flaxseed loaves:

Ingredients:

2 cups spelt flour.

1/2 cup ground flaxseed.

1 tablespoon of chia seeds.

1 teaspoon of baking soda.

1/2 teaspoon of salt.

1 cup of warm water.

1/4 cup honey.

1 tablespoon of olive oil.

1/4 cup of chopped walnuts (optional).

Instructions:

Preheat the oven to 350°F (175°C). Grease the loaf pan.

In a large bowl, whisk together spelt flour, ground flaxseed, chia seeds, baking soda, and salt.

In a separate bowl, whisk together warm water, honey, and olive oil.

Mix the wet ingredients with the dry ingredients until just combined. Fold in the chopped walnuts (if using).

Pour the batter into the prepared loaf pan. Bake for 50–60 minutes, or until a toothpick inserted in the centre comes out clean.

Allow the loaf to cool in its pan for 10 minutes before transferring it to a wire rack to finish cooling.

Slice, and enjoy!

Tips:

You can use other chopped nuts or seeds instead of walnuts.

For a sweeter bread, add an extra tablespoon of honey.

You can also make this bread in muffin tins for individual servings. Bake for 20-25 minutes, until golden brown and a toothpick inserted in the centre comes out clean.

4. Millet & Amaranth Bread:

Ingredients:

1 cup millet flour.

1/2 cup amaranth flour.

1/4 cup tapioca flour.

1 teaspoon of baking powder.

1/2 teaspoon of salt.

1 1/4 cups warm water.

1 tablespoon of olive oil.

One tablespoon honey (optional)

Instructions:

Preheat the oven to 375° Fahrenheit (190° Celsius).

Grease the loaf pan.

In a large mixing bowl, combine millet flour, amaranth flour, tapioca flour, baking powder, and salt.

In a separate mixing bowl, combine warm water, olive oil, and honey (if using).

Mix the wet ingredients with the dry ingredients until just combined. The dough will feel little sticky.

Pour the batter into the prepared loaf pan.

Bake for 50–60 minutes, or until a toothpick inserted in the centre comes out clean.

Allow the loaf to cool in its pan for 10 minutes before transferring it to a wire rack to finish cooling.

Slice, and enjoy!

Tips:

You can replace the millet and amaranth flours with other gluten-free flours, such as oat or almond flour.

To make a denser bread, add 1/4 cup ground flaxseed to the batter.

You can also make this bread in muffin tins for individual servings. Bake for 25 to 30 minutes, or until golden brown and a toothpick inserted in the centre comes out clean.

5. Chia seed flatbread:
Ingredients:
1/4 cup chia seeds.
1 cup water.
1 cup of all-purpose flour (or gluten-free flour blend).
1/2 teaspoon of baking powder.
1/4 teaspoon salt.
1 tablespoon of olive oil.

Instructions:
In a small bowl, mix the chia seeds and water. Set aside for 10 minutes, or until the mixture thickens and gels (chia pudding).
In a large bowl, combine the flour, baking powder, and salt.
Add the chia pudding and olive oil to the dry ingredients and combine until a dough forms.
Knead the dough on a lightly floured surface for a few minutes, or until smooth.
Divide the dough into four equal pieces. Roll out each piece to a thin circle.

Cook in a lightly greased griddle or frying pan over medium heat. Cook the flatbreads for 2-3 minutes on each side, or until golden brown and cooked through. Serve warm with your preferred toppings, such as hummus and vegetables, salsa and avocado, or nut butter and fruit.

Tips:

For added flavour, mix 1/4 cup chopped herbs or spices into the dough.

If the dough is too sticky, add a tablespoon of flour at a time until it is the right consistency.

You can also bake the flatbreads in a preheated oven at 400°F (200°C) for 10-12 minutes per side.

6. Brown Rice Tortilla:

Ingredients:

1 cup of cooked brown rice.

1/2 cup of warm water.

1/4 cup all-purpose flour (or gluten-free flour mixture)

1/4 teaspoon salt.

1 tablespoon of olive oil.

Instructions:

In a food processor, combine cooked brown rice and warm water until smooth.

Transfer the mixture to a bowl and mix in the flour, salt, and olive oil.

Knead for a few minutes until the dough is smooth and elastic.

Divide the dough into six equal pieces. Roll out each piece to a thin circle.

Cook in a lightly greased griddle or frying pan over medium heat. Cook the tortillas for 1-2 minutes on each side, or until golden brown and cooked through.

Serve warm with your preferred fillings, such as tacos, burritos, or enchiladas.

Tips:

For a Mexican-inspired flavour, mix 1/4 teaspoon chilli powder or cumin into the dough.

If the dough is too dry, add a tablespoon of water at a time until it is the right consistency.

You can also cook the tortillas in a preheated oven at 400°F (200°C) for 5-7 minutes on each side.

7. Quinoa and Black Bean Wrap:

Ingredients:

1 cup cooked quinoa.

1/2 cup cooked black beans, rinsed and drained

1/4 cup diced red onion

1/4 cup chopped green bell pepper.

1/4 cup chopped fresh cilantro.

1 tablespoon of lime juice.
1 tablespoon of olive oil.
1/2 teaspoon of chilli powder.
1/4 teaspoon cumin.
Pinch of salt and pepper, to taste.
Four large, whole wheat tortillas

Instructions:
In a large mixing bowl, combine cooked quinoa, black beans, red onion, green bell pepper, and cilantro.
In a small mixing bowl, combine the lime juice, olive oil, chilli powder, cumin, salt, and pepper.
Toss the dressing into the quinoa and black bean mixture.
Warm the tortillas in a microwave or dry skillet for about 30 seconds on each side.
Divide the black bean and quinoa mixture between the tortillas.
Roll the tortillas and enjoy!

Tips:
This recipe can be adapted to include other vegetables such as corn, chopped tomatoes, or avocado.
To add a spicy kick to the dressing, sprinkle with cayenne pepper or chopped jalapeno.

Feel free to use a variety of beans, such as pinto or kidney beans.

If you don't have cooked quinoa or black beans on hand, you can substitute canned or frozen versions. Just make sure you drain and rinse them thoroughly before using.

8. Cauliflower Pizza Crust:

Ingredients:

1 medium head of cauliflower, florets only (about 8 cups).

One egg, beaten

1/2 cup shredded mozzarella cheese.

1/4 cup grated parmesan cheese.

1 1/2 tablespoons coconut flour.

1/2 teaspoon of garlic powder.

1/2 teaspoon of dried oregano.

1/4 teaspoon salt.

Add freshly ground black pepper to taste.

Toppings of your choosing (pizza sauce, cheese, vegetables, etc.)

Instructions:

Preheat the oven to 425° Fahrenheit (220° Celsius).

Line a baking sheet with parchment paper.

Process the cauliflower florets in a food processor until they resemble rice. Place the riced cauliflower in a clean kitchen towel and squeeze out any excess moisture.

In a large bowl, combine the cauliflower rice, beaten egg, mozzarella, Parmesan, coconut flour, garlic powder, oregano, salt, and pepper. Mix thoroughly until combined.

Spread the cauliflower mixture evenly on the prepared baking sheet, forming a circular crust about 1/2 inch thick. Bake for 15-20 minutes, or until the crust turns golden brown and firm.

Remove the crust from the oven and add your preferred pizza toppings. Bake for an additional 10-15 minutes, or until the cheese melts and bubbles. Slice, and enjoy!

Tips:

To make a chewier crust, add 1/4 cup almond or chickpea flour to the mixture.

To save time, consider using pre-riced cauliflower.

Do not overcook the crust, as it will become dry and crumbly.

9. Gluten-free corn tortillas:

Ingredients:

1 cup of masa harina (corn flour).

1/2 teaspoon of salt.

1 1/4 cups warm water.

1 tablespoon of vegetable oil.

Instructions:
In a large mixing bowl, combine masa harina and salt.
Gradually add the warm water while stirring constantly until a soft dough forms. If the dough is too dry, add more water, one tablespoon at a time.
Knead for a few minutes until the dough is smooth.
Divide the dough into eight equal pieces. Roll each piece into a thin circle 6 inches in diameter.
Cook in a lightly greased griddle or frying pan over medium heat. Cook the tortillas for 1-2 minutes on each side, or until golden brown and cooked through.
Serve warm with your preferred fillings, such as tacos, burritos, or enchiladas.

Tips:
If you do not have masa harina, you can substitute a gluten-free all-purpose flour blend. However, the tortillas may not be as soft or pliable.
For a Mexican-inspired flavour, mix 1/4 teaspoon chilli powder or cumin into the dough.
If the dough is too sticky, add a tablespoon of masa harina at a time until it is the right consistency.

10. Buckwheat pancakes:

Ingredients:

1 cup buckwheat flour.

1/2 cup all-purpose flour (or any other gluten-free flour blend)

2 eggs

1 1/4 cup milk

1/4 teaspoon salt.

2 tablespoons melted butter.

Filling of your choosing (sweet or savoury)

Instructions:

In a large bowl, combine the buckwheat flour, all-purpose flour, eggs, milk, and salt.

Slowly whisk in the melted butter until the batter is completely smooth.

Place a lightly greased pancake pan or skillet over medium heat.

Pour about 1/4 cup batter into the pan and swirl to evenly coat the bottom.

Cook for 1-2 minutes on each side, or until the edges are golden brown and the centre is set.

Flip the pancake and cook for another 30 seconds.

Slide the pancake onto a plate and fill with your preferred filling. Fold or roll the pancake and enjoy!

Tips:

To make sweet crepes, add a tablespoon of sugar to the batter.

Savoury crepes should be filled with something savoury, such as cheese, vegetables, or meat.

If the crepes are sticking to the pan, turn down the heat slightly or add a little more butter.

Delicious Desserts and Sugar-Free Treats

1. Chocolate avocado mousse:

Ingredients:

Two ripe avocados, peeled and pitted.

1/4 cup cocoa powder.

1/4 cup maple syrup or honey

1/4 cup unsweetened almond or dairy milk

1 teaspoon of vanilla extract.

Pinch of salt.

Instructions:

In a food processor, puree the avocados until smooth and creamy.

Combine cocoa powder, maple syrup, almond milk, vanilla extract, and salt. Blend until well combined and the mixture reaches a mousse-like consistency.

Taste and adjust the sweetness or flavour as desired. You can add more cocoa powder for a richer chocolate flavour or more maple syrup for extra sweetness.

Divide the mousse among serving cups or glasses. Refrigerate for at least 30 minutes to allow it to set before serving.

Tips:

To make a thicker mousse, add a frozen banana or 1/4 cup frozen spinach to your blender.

To add flair, garnish the mousse with fresh berries, whipped cream, or shaved chocolate.

This mousse can be stored in the refrigerator for up to 2 days.

2. Creamy Coconut Ice Cream:

Ingredients:

2 cans (13.5 oz each) full-fat coconut milk, chilled overnight

1/4 cup maple syrup or honey

1 teaspoon of vanilla extract.

Pinch of salt.

Instructions:

Open the cans of coconut milk and scoop out the thick cream that has risen to the top, leaving the watery liquid behind. You should have about 2 cups of coconut cream.

Whip the coconut cream in a large bowl with an electric or stand mixer until stiff peaks form.

Add the maple syrup, vanilla extract, and salt, and continue mixing until everything is well combined.

Pour the mixture into a loaf pan or other freezer-safe container. Cover with plastic wrap and freeze for at least 4 hours, or until firm.
Let the ice cream soften slightly before scooping and serving.

Tips:
For a richer flavor, you can use full-fat coconut milk instead of light coconut milk.
Add 1/4 cup of chopped nuts or chocolate chips to the mixture for extra texture and flavor.
This ice cream can be stored in the freezer for up to 2 weeks.

3. Raw Chocolate Bark with Goji Berries:
Ingredients:
1 cup of melted dark chocolate (at least 70% cocoa).
1/2 cup chopped nuts (such as almonds, cashews, or peanuts)
1/4 cup dried goji berries.

Instructions:
Line a baking sheet with parchment paper.
Pour the melted chocolate onto the prepared baking sheet and spread it evenly into a thin layer.
Sprinkle the chopped nuts and goji berries over the chocolate.

Refrigerate for at least 30 minutes, or until the chocolate has set.

Break the bark into pieces and enjoy!

Tips:

You can substitute other dried fruits or nuts for goji berries.

For a fun twist, try adding a sprinkle of sea salt or cayenne pepper to the chocolate before refrigerating.

This bark can be stored in the refrigerator for up to a week.

4. Vanilla Bean Nice Cream:

Ingredients:

2 frozen bananas, peeled and chopped

1/2 cup milk (dairy or plant-based)

1/2 vanilla bean, seeds scraped out

One tablespoon honey (optional)

Pinch of sea salt (optional)

Instructions:

Add the frozen bananas, milk, and vanilla bean seeds to a high-powered blender or food processor.

Blend until smooth and creamy, scraping down the sides as required.

Taste and add honey or sea salt if desired.

Serve immediately for a soft-serve consistency, or transfer to an airtight container and freeze for 30-60 minutes for a harder scoop.

Tips:
For added flavor, add a spoonful of cocoa powder, peanut butter, or chopped nuts.
Use ripe bananas for the finest flavor.
You can use other frozen fruits like strawberries, mangoes, or pineapple for some of the bananas.

5. Strawberries and Cream Parfait:
Ingredients:
1 cup sliced fresh strawberries
1/2 cup plain yogurt (dairy or plant-based)
1/4 cup granola.
One tablespoon honey (optional)
Mint leaves for garnish (optional)

Instructions:
Layer the strawberries, yogurt, and granola in a parfait glass or mason jar.
Drizzle with honey if desired.
Garnish with fresh mint leaves (optional).

Tips:
Use other fruits like blueberries, raspberries, or peaches instead of strawberries.
For a richer flavor, use whipped cream instead of yogurt.
Make it a tiered parfait by alternating the fruit, yogurt, and granola layers.

6. Raw Key Lime Pie:
Ingredients:
Crust:
1 cup of pitted Medjool dates
1/2 cup unsweetened shredded coconut
1/4 cup raw almonds
1 tablespoon raw cacao powder (optional)

Filling:
1 cup soaked cashews, drained and rinsed
1/2 cup fresh lime juice
1/4 cup agave nectar or maple syrup
1/4 cup avocado oil
1 tablespoon lime zest
1/4 teaspoon sea salt

Instructions:
Crust:

Process the dates, coconut, nuts, and cacao powder (if using) in a food processor until crumbly.
Press the mixture into the bottom of a pie dish or springform pan.

Filling:
Blend the cashews, lime juice, agave nectar, avocado oil, lime zest, and sea salt in a high-powered blender until smooth and creamy.
Pour the filling onto the crust.
Freeze for at least 4 hours, or until set.

Tips:
Use a blender with high blending power for a smooth filling.
Soak the cashews for at least 4 hours, preferably overnight, for a creamier filling.
Garnish the pie with sliced limes, coconut flakes, or fresh mint leaves.

7. Sugar-Free Chocolate Truffles:
Ingredients:
1 cup of pitted Medjool dates
1/4 cup unsweetened cocoa powder.
1/4 cup almond butter
1 tablespoon coconut oil, melted
1/4 teaspoon of vanilla extract.

A pinch of sea salt.

Instructions:
Process the dates in a food processor until finely ground.
Add the cocoa powder, almond butter, melted coconut oil, vanilla extract, and salt.
Blend until smooth and sticky.
Roll the ingredients into little balls using your hands.
Roll the truffles in additional cocoa powder, chopped almonds, or shredded coconut (optional).
Store the truffles in an airtight jar in the refrigerator for up to a week.

Tips:
If the mixture is too dry, add a tablespoon of water or melted coconut oil.
Use several varieties of nut butter for varied flavor variations.
Roll the truffles with edible glitter for a festive touch.

8. Skillet Apple Crisp:
Ingredients:
For the filling:
4-5 apples (approximately 2 pounds), peeled, cored, and sliced
1/4 cup granulated sugar.

2 teaspoons brown sugar
1 tablespoon cornstarch
Half a teaspoon of crushed cinnamon
Pinch of salt.

For the topping:
1/2 cup rolled oats.
1/4 cup all-purpose flour
1/4 cup light brown sugar
1/4 cup chopped pecans or walnuts
1/4 cup cold, unsalted butter, cubed
1/4 teaspoon of ground cinnamon.
Pinch of salt.

Instructions:
Preheat the oven to 375° Fahrenheit (190° Celsius). Prepare a cast-iron pan by lightly coating it with butter.
In a large bowl, combine the sliced apples, granulated sugar, brown sugar, cornstarch, cinnamon, and salt. Toss to coat the apples evenly.
Transfer the apple mixture to the preheated skillet.
In a separate bowl, combine the oats, flour, brown sugar, almonds, chilled butter, cinnamon, and salt. Using your fingertips or a pastry cutter, combine the ingredients together until you have a crumbly mixture.

Sprinkle the crumb topping evenly over the apple filling.

Bake for 30-35 minutes, or until the apples are soft and the topping is golden brown.

Allow to cool slightly before serving. Enjoy warm with a spoonful of vanilla ice cream or whipped cream (optional).

Tips:

You can use other types of apples, such as Granny Smith, Gala, or Honeycrisp.

For a streusel topping, use a fork to form larger clumps of the topping before dusting over the apples. Add 1/4 cup dried cranberries or raisins to the topping for added flavor.

9. Low-Carb Cheesecake Bites:

Ingredients:

For the crust:

1/2 cup almond flour

1/4 cup melted coconut oil.

1 tablespoon honey.

Pinch of salt.

For the filling:

1/2 cup cream cheese, softened

1/4 cup of unsweetened almond milk.

1 tablespoon of lemon juice.

1 tablespoon honey.

1/4 teaspoon of vanilla extract.

Pinch of salt.

Instructions:

Preheat the oven to 350°F (175°C). Prepare a muffin tray by lining it with paper liners.

In a small mixing dish, add almond flour, melted coconut oil, honey, and salt. Mix well until a crumbly dough forms.

Press the dough into the bottom of each muffin cup, producing a tiny crust.

In a separate dish, mix together the softened cream cheese, almond milk, lemon juice, honey, vanilla essence, and salt until smooth.

Fill each muffin cup with the cheesecake filling.

Bake for 15-20 minutes, or until the filling is set.

Let cool entirely in the pan before transferring to a wire rack to cool further.

Refrigerate in an airtight container for up to three days.

Tips:

You can use a little muffin tray to produce smaller bits.

Top the cheesecake bits with fresh berries, whipped cream, or a sprinkle of sugar-free chocolate chips before serving.
For a deeper flavor, use full-fat cream cheese.

10. Caramelized Pear Upside Down Cake
Ingredients:
For the caramelized pears:
4 ripe pears, peeled, cored, and halved
1/4 cup unsalted butter
1/4 cup brown sugar
1 tablespoon water
1/4 teaspoon of ground cinnamon.
Pinch of salt.

For the cake:
1 1/2 cups all-purpose flour.
1 teaspoon of baking powder.
1/2 teaspoon of baking soda.
1/4 teaspoon salt.
1/2 cup unsalted butter, softened.
1 cup granulated sugar.
Two huge eggs.
1 teaspoon of vanilla extract.
1 cup buttermilk

Instructions:

Preheat the oven to 375° Fahrenheit (190° Celsius). Butter a 9-inch round cake pan.

In a large saucepan, melt the butter over medium heat. Add the brown sugar, water, cinnamon, and salt. Bring to a boil and cook, stirring periodically, for 5-7 minutes, or until the sugar dissolves and the sauce thickens slightly.

Arrange the pear halves in the prepared cake pan, cut side down, in a circular pattern or whatever you wish. Pour the warm caramel sauce over the pears.

In a large bowl, whisk together the flour, baking powder, baking soda, and salt.

In a separate dish, mix together the softened butter and sugar until light and fluffy. Beat in the eggs one at a time, then stir in the vanilla essence.

Alternately add the dry ingredients and buttermilk to the wet components, mixing just until blended. Don't overmix.

Pour the cake batter over the caramelized pears in the pan. Smooth the top with a spatula.

Bake for 40-45 minutes, or until a toothpick inserted into the center comes out clean.

Let the cake cool in the pan for 10 minutes before inverting it onto a plate. Serve warm with a scoop of vanilla ice cream or whipped cream (optional).

Tips:

For a deeper caramel flavor, use dark brown sugar instead of light brown sugar.

You can add 1/2 cup chopped nuts to the cake batter for extra texture.

If you don't have buttermilk, you can make your own by adding 1 tablespoon of lemon juice or vinegar to 1 cup of milk and letting it sit for 5 minutes.

Chapter 3: Personalized Approach to Baking

As you embark upon your journey towards lymph-friendly baking, personalization becomes a critical aspect of crafting delectable creations that cater to unique dietary needs, allergies, sensitivities, and preferences. In this chapter, we delve deeper into customizing recipes according to individual requirements, allowing you to enjoy wholesome baked goods tailor-made for your lifestyle and wellbeing goals.

Tailoring Recipes to Unique Dietary Needs

Recognizing that everyone's nutritional demands varies, adopting a tailored approach to baking helps you to fulfil various dietary needs. Consider the following scenarios:

1. Gluten-Free: Individuals with celiac disease or non-celiac gluten sensitivity must avoid wheat, barley, and rye products. By replacing conventional flours with gluten-free alternatives, such as rice flour, sorghum flour, or almond flour, you can accommodate gluten-free diets.

2. Dairy-Free: Those who are lactose intolerant or follow a vegan diet should opt for dairy-free alternatives, such as almond milk, soy milk, or coconut milk. You might also consider using vegan butter or coconut oil in place of conventional butter.

3. Low-FODMAP: People having irritable bowel syndrome (IBS) or other digestive disorders may find relief by restricting Fermentable Oligosaccharides, Disaccharides, Monosaccharides, And Polyols (FODMAPs), a category of short-chain carbohydrates. By omitting high-FODMAP ingredients, such as garlic, onion, and wheat, you may create low-FODMAP versions of your favorite baked products.

4. Keto-Friendly: If you follow a ketogenic diet, favour low-carbohydrate, moderate-protein, and high-fat products, such as coconut flour, almond flour, and avocado oil. Avoid high-glycemic index ingredients, such as sugar and white flour.

5. Paleo-Friendly: The paleolithic diet emphasizes consuming complete, unprocessed foods similar to what early humans ate throughout the Paleolithic era. By excluding grains, legumes, dairy, and processed foods, you can create paleo-friendly baked goods featuring ingredients like coconut flour, arrowroot powder, and grass-fed gelatin.

Adapting for Allergies and Sensitivities

Allergies and sensitivities can cause issues when it comes to baking. However, by carefully evaluating probable triggers, you can alter recipes properly.

Below are common allergy and sensitivity adaptations:

1. Tree Nut Allergies: Eliminate tree nuts, such as almonds, hazelnuts, and pistachios, and replace them with seed-based alternatives, such as sunflower seeds or pumpkin seeds.

2. Peanut Allergies: Exclude peanuts and use alternate legume flours, such as garbanzo bean flour or black bean flour, or substitute with sunflower seed butter or tiger nut butter.

3. Seafood Allergies: Remove shellfish and fish from recipes and utilize alternate animal proteins, such as chicken or beef, or plant-based proteins, such as tofu or tempeh.

4. Shellfish Allergies: Eliminate shellfish and explore with other animal proteins, such as chicken or beef, or plant-based proteins, such as tofu or tempeh.

5. Egg Allergies: Replace eggs with egg alternatives, such as flaxseed gel, aquafaba, or commercial egg replacement powders.

6. Soy Allergies: Minimize soy consumption by choosing soy-free alternatives, such as almond milk, coconut milk, or hemp milk, and select soy-free flours, such as almond flour or buckwheat flour.

Customizing for Preferences and Tastes

Individual tastes and inclinations play a vital influence in deciding the success of your baking attempts. By taking into account personal likes and dislikes, you can ensure that every bite is deliciously rewarding. Consider the following tips:

1. Flavor Variations: Introduce different flavors by adding fresh herbs, spices, extracts, or citrus zests to your dishes. For example, try adding lemon zest to a vanilla loaf or cinnamon to a chocolate chip cookie recipe.

2. Texture Modifications: Adjust texture by adjusting the consistency of your dough or batter. For instance, add rolled oats to muffins for added chewiness or increase the amount of psyllium husk in bread to obtain a denser texture.

3. Sweetener Alternatives: Explore several types of sweeteners to suit your palette. Natural sweeteners, such as maple syrup, agave nectar, or monk fruit extract, offer varied levels of sweetness and flavor characteristics.

4. Fat Content: Manage the fat content of your baked goods by altering the type and quantity of fats used. For example, switch half of the butter in a recipe with Greek yogurt or apple sauce to lessen total fat intake.

5. Portion Control: Ensure portion control by splitting your baked products into smaller servings. For instance, cut giant cookies into quarters or slice brownies into smaller pieces to restrict serving size.

By embracing a tailored approach to baking, you can confidently traverse the world of lymph-friendly cuisine, addressing various dietary needs, allergies, sensitivities, and preferences. As your knowledge and talents grow, you'll uncover countless chances to produce delightful and healthful baked items that are suited to your unique wellness goals.

Chapter 4: Tips for Culinary Exploration and Self-Discovery

Embarking on a journey toward lymph-friendly baking isn't just about learning recipes and improving technique—it's also about fostering awareness, enjoying the process, and building supporting groups along the way.

Mindful Eating Practices

Mindful eating fosters awareness and appreciation of the food you consume, building a positive relationship between your body and the food you eat. Implementing mindful eating activities can improve your general health and strengthen your connection to lymph-friendly cuisine.

Here are some ways to practice mindfulness eating:

1. Slowing Down: Take time to taste each bite, rather than hurrying through meals. Slow down to appreciate the textures, scents, and flavors of your lymph-friendly baked goodies.

2. Listening to Your Body: Pay attention to hunger and fullness signals, acknowledging your body's need for nourishment and satisfaction. Respect your appetite and quit eating once you are satiated.

3. Being current: Engage all five senses when eating, focusing entirely on the current moment. Notice how the food looks, smells, feels, and tastes.

4. Reducing Distractions: Turn off electronic gadgets and eliminate distractions during eating. Create a tranquil environment favorable to mindful eating.

5. Showing Gratitude: Express gratitude for the food you make and consume. Reflect on the labor and care that went into creating your lymph-friendly baked goodies.

Enjoying the Journey of Cooking

Accepting the joy and fulfilment inherent in the process of cooking will help you turn your baking adventures into gratifying voyages of discovery and progress. Here are some strategies to make the most of your time spent in the kitchen:

1. **Experimenting with New Techniques:** Try unique baking processes and techniques to widen your skill set and challenge yourself artistically.

2. **Exploring Different Cuisines:** Expand your repertoire by learning about and trying recipes from various cultures and areas around the globe.

3. **Using Seasonal food**: Integrate seasonal food into your baking practice to take advantage of fresh, locally produced ingredients.

4. Working with Friends and Family: Invite loved ones to join you in the kitchen, where you can share ideas, techniques, and laughs while creating lymph-friendly baked treats.

5. Documenting Your Progress: Keep track of your baking accomplishments and progress by photographing your creations, writing about your experiences, or sharing your stories online.

Sharing with Others and Forming a Supportive Community

Sharing your enthusiasm for lymph-friendly baking with others can help you build relationships, encourage creativity, and reinforce your dedication to healthy living. Here are several ways to share your passion for lymph-friendly baking with friends, family, and other enthusiasts:

1. Hosting Social Events: Plan parties centred on lymph-friendly baking, asking others to sample your creations and learn about the benefits of lymph-friendly cuisine.

2. Joining Online Communities: Connect with like-minded folks through social media groups, blogs, and forums focused on lymph-friendly baking and wellbeing. Share recipes, insights, and advice with people following similar interests.

3. Attending Local Workshops and seminars: Join local workshops and seminars conducted by qualified instructors to enhance your baking abilities and meet other bakers.

4. Volunteering at Charitable Organizations: Donate your time and knowledge to charitable organizations that help persons with lymphedema and lipedema. Teach basic baking skills and provide lymph-friendly recipes to those in need.

5. Giving Back to the Community: Participate in community initiatives that raise awareness about lymphedema and lipedema, such as fundraising events, educational programmes, and advocacy campaigns.

By embracing mindful eating practices, enjoying the process of cooking, and sharing your love with others, you may open up a world of culinary inquiry and self-discovery. As you immerse yourself in the world of lymph-friendly baking, remember to enjoy your triumphs, treasure the moments of creativity, and recognise the power of community.

Conclusion

By the end of this guide, you'll have a better awareness of the fundamentals of lymph-friendly baking, personalized approaches to recipe adaptation, and tips for culinary exploration and self-discovery. By taking a holistic approach to lymphatic health, you can create tasty and nourishing baked items that will help you achieve your wellness objectives and improve your quality of life.

Throughout this guide, we've covered numerous fundamental concepts for lymph-friendly baking, including:

1. The fundamentals of a lymph-friendly diet, including complete foods, balanced macronutrients, and appropriate hydration.

2. Key elements for lymphedema and lipedema include leafy green vegetables, cruciferous vegetables, antioxidant-rich fruits, omega-3 fatty acids, probiotic-rich fermented meals, plant-based proteins, and prebiotic fibres.

3. Healthy baking alternatives include substituting white flour with whole grain flours, using unsweetened applesauce instead of butter or oil, and experimenting with different milks and sweeteners.

4. Personalised techniques to recipe adaptation, such as modifying recipes to specific nutritional requirements, adjusting for allergies and sensitivities, and customising for preferences and tastes.

5. Tips for culinary research and self-discovery include mindful eating, appreciating the process of cooking, sharing with others, and forming a supportive community.

As you continue your culinary journey towards lymph-friendly baking, remember to approach it with inquiry, creativity, and compassion. Embrace the joy and fulfilment that cooking brings, and celebrate your accomplishments along the way. Whether you're trying new skills, discovering new cuisines, or sharing your enthusiasm with others, you can be confident that you're improving your health and wellbeing.

By introducing lymph-friendly baking into your daily routine, you may actively manage lymphedema and lipedema, promote healthy lymphatic function, and improve your overall quality of life. So, go ahead and enjoy the benefits of lymph-friendly baking, as well as the tasty and nutritious products that await you.

www.ingramcontent.com/pod-product-compliance
Lightning Source LLC
Chambersburg PA
CBHW070812260726
48660CB00005B/1830